I0845441

Things to consider while expecting:

A First-Time Guide to a Healthier Pregnancy Journey From Wellness Practices to Useful Planning

By

Darla B Humphrey

Copyright :

© (2023) by [**Darla B. Humphrey**]

Protected by copyright law. No piece of this distribution might be duplicated, circulated, or communicated in any structure or using any and all means, including copying, recording, or other electronic or mechanical techniques, without the earlier consent of the distributer, with the exception of brief citations epitomised in basic audits and certain other noncommercial purposes allowed by intellectual property regulation.

Disclaimer:

The data given in this [**Things to consider while expecting**] is for general enlightening purposes as it were. It isn't expected to fill in for proficient clinical, legal, or monetary counsel. Perusers are urged to talk with proper experts for exhortations customised to their singular conditions.

The writer and distributor make no representations or guarantees with respect to the precision, fulfilment, or reasonableness of the data contained

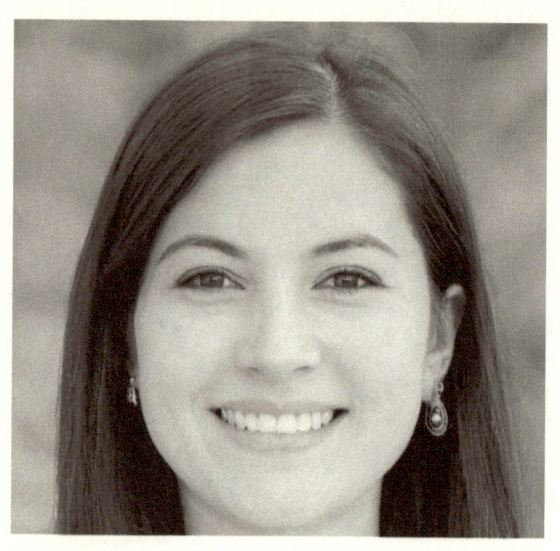

About the author

Darla B. Humphrey is a devoted creator with a foundation in nursing, zeroing in on giving common-sense experiences to eager moms. Her work probably revolves around tending to the different parts of pregnancy, offering direction, and assisting ladies with exploring the excursion to parenthood. By consolidating her nursing mastery enthusiastically for supporting eager moms, Humphrey means to engage ladies with important data and assets during this extraordinary time of their lives.

While explicit insights concerning Darla B. Humphrey's life and vocation might require a more top-to-bottom examination, her obligation to support eager moms recommends a merciful and educated approach. It's plausible that her compositions dive into themes like pre-birth care, labor readiness, post-pregnancy prosperity, and perhaps even infant care. Humphrey probably draws from her nursing experience to offer proof-based guidance, encouraging a feeling of certainty and readiness for moms-to-be as they explore the difficulties and delights of pregnancy. For a complete comprehension of her work, investigating her distributed books, articles, or any suitable meetings would give further bits of knowledge into her commitments to maternal wellbeing.

Bonus.

Knowing the warning signs and symptoms of issues that arise after delivery

INTRODUCTION

CHAPTER 1

Preparation for a healthy pregnancy:

Planning for pregnancy and lifestyle adjustments

Types of pregnancy

Chapter2

Nutritional Guidelines:

Nutritional Essentials for You and Baby

Chapter 3:

Safety Guidelines : Do's and Don'ts

Do's During Pregnancy:

Don'ts During Pregnancy:

Practical tips for a safe and healthy pregnancy

Nurturing a Healthy Pregnancy

Chapter4

Guiding Your Health Through Pregnancy:

Monitoring vital signs and addressing concerns

Common pregnancy symptoms and management

Exercise during pregnancy

Chapter 5:

Trimester Insights and Changes:

Understanding the Three Pregnancy Phases

Complications of pregnancy

Chapter 6

Labor and Delivery:

Final stages of pregnancy

Chapter 7

Postpartum Care:

Newborn care basics

Infant illnesses

Chapter 8

Emotional adjustment:

Recognizing postpartum depression and seeking support

Role of dad's in postpartum

Chapter 9

Parenting:

Parenting Tips and Advice:

Knowing the warning signs and symptoms of issues that arise after delivery

INTRODUCTION

Welcome to "Things to consider while expecting:A First-Time Guide to a Healthier Pregnancy Journey From Wellness Practices to Useful Planning

An aide was created with care for hopeful moms on the striking excursion to parenthood. Created by Darla B. Humphrey, a carefully prepared nurture energetic about maternal prosperity, this book is intended to give you down to earth and enable bits of knowledge as you cross the way of pregnancy.

Pregnancy is a significant and groundbreaking experience, and each expecting mother merits dependable data and direction to explore this section of life. "Things to Consider while expecting:A First-Time Guide to a Healthier Pregnancy Journey From Wellness Practices to Useful Planning "is something other than a book; it's a buddy offering proof-based exhortation, consistent encouragement, and an abundance of information gained from long periods of nursing experience.

Inside these pages, you'll track down an extensive and caring investigation of the groundbreaking journey of pregnancy. As you explore the unknown waters of eager parenthood, this book is intended to be your dependable buddy, offering bits of knowledge, guidance, and a consoling voice to go with you constantly.

Expecting your most memorable kid is a groundbreaking event loaded with expectation, marvel, and, indeed, a couple of vulnerabilities. Darla B. Humphrey, a sympathetic medical caretaker and creator, has woven together an embroidery of information, useful hints, and genuine support custom-made explicitly for first-time moms. Whether you're looking for direction on pre-birth care, wellbeing techniques, or conquering difficulties, this guide is here to engage you to settle on educated choices and embrace excellence regarding this one-of-a-kind section of your life.

Thus, we should set out on this thrilling excursion together, investigating the subtleties of sound pregnancy, developing health, and beating difficulties with flexibility. "

In these pages, you will track down an extensive investigation of pre-birth care, labor planning, and post-pregnancy contemplations, and that's just the beginning. From addressing normal worries to praising the delights of pregnancy, this book plans to equip you with the devices and information expected to settle on informed choices, encouraging a feeling of certainty and status.

Keep in mind that each pregnancy is special, and this book is definitely not a one-size-fits-all arrangement. It is an educational asset to supplement the individualised consideration you get from medical services experts. As you dive into the parts ahead, may you track down consolation, find significant bits of knowledge, and embrace the expectation and marvel that accompany anticipating another life.

Here's to a sound and cheerful excursion into parenthood. Inside these pages, Darla B. Humphrey joins her clinical mastery with a real comprehension of the close-to-home and actual parts of pregnancy. As a medical caretaker profoundly dedicated to maternal wellbeing, she perceives the requirement for hopeful moms to feel upheld, informed, and engaged during this groundbreaking period

CHAPTER 1

Preparation for a healthy pregnancy:

Planning for pregnancy and lifestyle adjustments

Here are a few fundamental tips to assist you with getting ready for this unique time in your life:

Throw your anti-conception medication:

Before you can imagine it, clearly, you need to quit taking your anti-conception medication. Be that as it may, it's generally not as basic as stopping and becoming pregnant the next week. You ought to follow the accompanying rules for halting anti-conception medication:

- Quit utilising oral contraceptives, NuvaRing, or the Fix two cycles before you need to get pregnant.
- Have an IUD eliminated a month prior.
- Let the last portion of injectable types of anti-conception medication, such as Depo-Provera, wear off 90 days before origination.

This will allow your chemical levels an opportunity to reset and will permit you to follow your period and realise when ovulation—the time you're probably going to get pregnant—happens. (You can likewise attempt an internet-based ovulation number cruncher.) All things considered, certain individuals get pregnant just subsequent to halting conception prevention. Continuously use boundary contraceptives so you don't get pregnant before you plan to.

Balance the scales:

Studies have shown that being underweight or overweight can influence richness and fetal wellbeing. For instance, research has observed that corpulence is related to an absence of ovulation.

Essentially, being underweight has been related to the following:

Diminished implantation rates

Diminished clinical pregnancy

Diminished continuous pregnancy

Chat with a medical care supplier to figure out your ideal weight and the steps you really want to take to arrive.

Resolve it:

Being truly dynamic before (and during) pregnancy has benefits. The more fit you are, the simpler your pregnancy and delivery might be.

You can proceed with your activity routine assuming you're now dynamic; simply be certain not to go overboard. Just before you imagine it isn't an ideal opportunity to prepare for a long-distance race or lift gigantic loads.

Make an effort not to push yourself unreasonably hard if you're basically beginning an activity program. Whether you're a health buff or a novice, look at your dynamic work with a clinical consideration provider to get the endorsement.

Avoid Caffeine:

Research suggests that caffeine doesn't appear to impact fertility. However, during pregnancy, an abundance of caffeine can incite unexpected labor or preterm birth.

That is the explanation the American School of Obstetricians and Gynecologists (ACOG) endorses for limiting caffeine in pregnancy to something like 200 milligrams every day (around one 12-ounce cup of coffee).

Regardless of the review, it's not just a coffee or tea thing: chocolate, soda pops, juiced refreshments, and some cold and torture solutions similarly have caffeine.

Avoid stress:

Stress can seemingly impact you for eternity. While endeavouring to envision, the American Culture for Regenerative Drugs (ASRM) says that tension reduces sexual respect, satisfaction, and the repeat of intercourse.

Cutting out the edge for yourself reliably and taking part in care practice can help you diminish strain.

Clean Up Your Eating Routine:

To get your pregnancy moving right, eat food assortments from all of the five nourishment types, which include:

- Natural items
- Vegetables

- Grains
- Lean proteins (like chicken, eggs, and beans)

Avoid food assortments high in fat and sugar, and guarantee you're getting a sufficient number of fluids. Carrying out dietary enhancements when you're still in the endeavouring-to-envision stage will get you ready for a more direct pregnancy diet makeover once you become pregnant and help you stay strong.

Take Mindfulness with Fish:

The U.S. Food and Drug Administration (FDA) suggests staying away from specific fish (swordfish, shark, lord mackerel, and tilefish) when pregnant as a result of their elevated levels of mercury. They say the best fish decisions are most reduced in mercury, yet even with these, you ought to restrict them to two times per week.

As indicated by the FDA, the best fish decisions
include:

- Anchovy
- Catfish
- Cod
- Crab
- Wallow
- Herring
- Lobster
- Shellfish
- Roost
- Salmon
- Sardines
- Shrimp
- Tilapia
- Trout

A lot of mercury can harm a hatchling's
developing cerebrum and sensory system.

Despite the fact that there is no particular suggestion for those who haven't yet considered it, It's smart to keep the rules for pregnancy so you'll, as of now, have this propensity set up.

Support Your Folate:

Enough folic corrosive can assist with preventing birth defects in a child's head and spine. Janis Biermann, MS, previous senior VP for instruction and wellbeing advancement at the Walk of Dimes, says getting 400 micrograms of folic corrosive consistently and eating high-folate food varieties is significant.

Most pre-birth nutrients ought to meet your day-to-day folate needs. Some great food hotspots for folic corrosive include:

- Verdant vegetables
- Beans
- Citrus organic products
- Entire grains
- Folate-enhanced cereals and bread

The CDC suggests increasing your folic corrosive admission one month prior to attempting to get pregnant.

Take Enhancements:

Notwithstanding folic corrosive, it's likewise really smart to guarantee you're getting an adequate number of different nutrients in your eating routine. A decent pre-birth nutrient is a superb method for doing so. These enhancements contain the fundamental nutrients needed to guarantee a sound pregnancy. Pre-birth nutrients include:

- Folic corrosive
- Iron
- Calcium
- Vitamin D
- L-ascorbic acid
- Iodine

Since you won't know you're pregnant immediately, taking a pre-birth nutrient while attempting to consider it can guarantee you have every one of the supplements prepared for when you are pregnant.

Quit Smoking:

As per the FDA, smoking while at the same time attempting to consider it can affect richness in the accompanying ways:

- Lessening ripeness
- Adversely influencing chemical creation

- Hurting the conceptual framework
- Harming the DNA in sperm

Likewise, when pregnant, smoking adversely influences the hatchling. Individuals who smoke during pregnancy are in danger of low birth weight, deficient lung advancement, preterm birth, or passing on an unexpected baby death condition (SIDS).

On the off chance that you smoke, quit—sooner, the better."

For smokers utilising discontinuance help, similar to nicotine gums or fixes or remedies like Zyban or Chantix, permit sufficient time for the medicine to work and afterward wean yourself off it for essentially a month prior to origination.

Stop Alcohol:

Since you'll be pregnant for essentially half a month in a flash, the CDC prompts anybody attempting to imagine to quit drinking. Liquor use in pregnancy can prompt unsuccessful labor and stillbirth.

Also, investigations have discovered that weighty drinking while at the same time attempting to get pregnant could make it more difficult to imagine. For instance, a recent report found that weighty consumers had diminished egg quality and a decreased likelihood of becoming pregnant in one monthly cycle.

Limit soda and natural product juice:

Investigations have discovered that drinking sugar-improved refreshments is related to decreased chances of pregnancy. Thus, it is presumably best to restrict soft drinks while attempting to consider.

It's likewise smart to wipe out trans fats from your eating regimen, as consuming an excess of them has been linked to fruitlessness. Specialists accept that trans fats influence regenerative wellbeing by diminishing egg quality.

See a medical services supplier:

Indeed, go through your rundown of medications, both prescription and over-the-counter, with your supplier to ensure not a single one of them would be unsafe for the pregnancy. " Remember to remember any home-grown enhancements and nutrients for the rundown.

Types of pregnancy

Pregnancy is a complex organic interaction of different sorts, each introducing interesting qualities and contemplations. The principal types include:

- . **Singleton pregnancy**

The most well-known type, where a lady conveys just a single hatchling,.

That is, a single-baby pregnancy at a time.

- **MultiplePregnancy**:

A multiple pregnancy is defined as a pregnancy involving multiple fetuses. Multiple eggs may implant and grow in the uterus if multiple eggs are released during the menstrual cycle and each egg is fertilized by a sperm.

- **Ectopic Pregnancy:**

When a fertilized egg implants itself outside of the womb, generally in one of the fallopian tubes, it is known as an ectopic pregnancy.it won't hatch into a baby and, should the pregnancy proceed, it could endanger your health.

- **Molar Pregnancy:**

Described by the strange development of trophoblastic cells, prompting the arrangement of a mass or growth.

Types incorporate total and incomplete molar pregnancies.

Generally non-feasible and requires clinical consideration.

- **Blighted ovum:**

A disorder that arises when an embryo fails to develop inside the gestational sac.

It happens when an embryo ceases to develop or never begins. Frequently, no clear cause is found. Usually, an ultrasound in the early weeks of pregnancy detects it. At the point when a gestational sac grows, yet the undeveloped organism doesn't. Frequently, it brings about an unnatural birth cycle and may require clinical administration.

- **Chemical Pregnancy:**

An early pregnancy misfortune that happens soon after implantation. A chemical pregnancy occurs when a woman miscarries very early, usually in the first five weeks of her pregnancy. An embryo develops, may even implant itself in the lining of your uterus (implantation), and then ceases to grow. Chemical pregnancies happen so early in life that many miscarry without realising it.

- **Cryptic pregnancy:**

It is an uncommon condition where a woman knows nothing about her pregnancy until late in the term. Can be trying to analyse because of negligible or missing pregnancy side effects.

- **High Risk Pregnancy** :

Pregnancy at high risk may be caused by a number of risk factors, including pre-existing medical disorders like diabetes, high blood pressure, or HIV positivity. obesity and overweight. High blood pressure, preeclampsia, gestational diabetes, stillbirth, neural tube abnormalities, and caesarean delivery are among the conditions that obesity raises the risk for.

Chapter2

Nutritional Guidelines:

Nutritional Essentials for You and Baby

Ensuring adequate nutrition is essential for you and your unborn child during pregnancy and beyond. In addition to a healthy diet, your healthcare provider might make specific recommendations for supplements, such as prenatal vitamins, to ensure you are meeting all your nutritional needs.

A balanced diet provides essential nutrients that support your child's growth and development while also maintaining your own health. Here's a thorough look at healthy fundamentals for both:

- Folic Corrosive (Folate): Prevents brain tube abandonment and is crucial for the early fetal course of events. Guarantee a sufficient admission of folate, a B-nutrient critical for brain tube improvement.Excellent sources include braced grains, beans, and mixed greens; green vegetables; sustained oats; and citrus organic products.

- Iron: Because pregnancy increases blood volume, more iron is needed to ensure adequate oxygen transport. Include vegetables, lean meats, and iron-braced foods to prevent illness. Your child's red platelet development and oxygen transport depend on iron in their diet.

- Calcium is essential for strengthening the child's and your own bones. Mixed greens, dairy products, and plant-based milk are excellent sources. Consolidate dairy items, strengthened plant-based milk, and salad greens into your eating regimen to meet your calcium needs. Calcium is imperative for the improvement of a child's bones and teeth.

- Protein: Important for the growth of cells. Include fish, poultry, eggs, dairy, vegetables, nuts, and lean meats in your diet. Vital for the development of the child's organs and tissues. Sufficient protein is fundamental for the development of the child's tissues. Incorporate lean meats, poultry, fish, eggs, dairy items, vegetables, and nuts into your dinners.

- Omega-3 unsaturated fats support the development of the child's mind and eyes. Pecans, chia seeds, flaxseeds, and greasy fish are excellent sources. Omega-3 unsaturated fats, especially DHA, are significant for the child's cerebrum and eye improvement. Consolidate greasy fish like salmon, chia seeds, flaxseeds, and pecans into your eating regimen.

- Iodine is important for thyroid function, which affects the mental health of the child. Good sources include dairy products, fish, and iodized salt.

- L-ascorbic acid strengthens the safe framework and enhances iron retention. Broccoli, ringer peppers, strawberries, and organic citrus products are rich sources of L-ascorbic acid.

- Fibre: Include high-fibre foods in your diet, such as whole grains, organic products, vegetables, and fruits, to help prevent clogging, which is common during pregnancy.

- Hydration: It's critical that you and your child stay adequately hydrated. Water prevents drying out and plays a fundamental role in many physical processes.

- Vitamin A is important for the development of the child's vision and resistant framework. Add sources such as dull salad greens, carrots, and yams.

- Vitamin E promotes the growth of the child's cells. Excellent sources are nuts, seeds, and vegetable oils.

- Vitamin K is essential to thickening the blood. Vitamin K is found in certain oils and in green, leafy vegetables.

- Vitamin D aids in the absorption of calcium for healthy bones. Spend your energy outside and include sources such as plant or dairy milk and fatty fish.

Chapter 3:

Safety Guidelines : Do's and Don'ts

Do's During Pregnancy:

- Go to Customary Pre-birth Check-ups:

Plan and go to all suggested pre-birth check-ups. These arrangements are urgent for checking both your wellbeing and the child's turn of events.

- Keep a Reasonable Eating Routine:

Focus on organic products, vegetables, entire grains, lean proteins, and dairy to help the child's development.

- Take part in moderate activity.

Take part in ordinary, moderate activity with your medical care supplier's endorsement. Exercises like strolling, swimming, and pre-birth yoga can generally advance prosperity.

- Get Satisfactory Rest:

Guarantee that you get sufficient rest. Pay attention to your body's signs and enjoy reprieves when expected to oversee weakness and decrease pressure.

- Remain Hydrated:

Drink a lot of water to remain hydrated. Legitimate hydration is fundamental for keeping up with amniotic fluid levels and supporting large-scale wellbeing.

- Teach Yourself:

Find out about the various phases of pregnancy, labor, and postpartum care. Go to pre-birth classes to acquire significant information and plan for the impending changes.

- Practise great cleanliness.

Keep up with great individual cleanliness by cleaning up routinely. This diminishes the risk of diseases that can influence both you and the child.

- Wear Open to Attire:

Decide on a dress that suits your evolving body. Strong shoes can ease distress and decrease stress on your back and feet.

Keep in mind that each pregnancy is one of a kind, so it's critical to tailor these do's to your singular necessities. Standard correspondence with your medical services supplier guarantees customised direction and a smoother pregnancy venture.

Don'ts During Pregnancy:

- Stay away from liquor and tobacco.

Avoid liquor and tobacco items. Both can present serious dangers to the child, influencing their development and advancement.

- Limit Caffeine Admission:

While moderate caffeine utilization is for the most part viewed as protected, inordinate admission ought to be avoided. Limit your day-to-day caffeine intake to lessen your expected chances.

- Be Wary of Prescriptions:Counsel your medical services supplier prior to taking any prescriptions, including non-prescription medications. A few drugs might have unfavourable impacts during pregnancy.

- Keep away from specific food sources:

Avoid crude or half-cooked fish, eggs, and meats to limit the risk of foodborne illnesses. Additionally, stay away from unpasteurized dairy items.

- Limit openness to destructive synthetic compounds:

Be wary of your openness to synthetic compounds, pesticides, and cleaning specialists. Guarantee great ventilation while utilising family items to diminish inward breath chances.

- Limit Fish High in Mercury:Stay away from fish with high mercury levels, like sharks, swordfish, lord mackerel, and tilefish. Select low-mercury choices like salmon, trout, and shrimp.

- Stay away from hot tubs and saunas.

Delayed openness to high temperatures, like hot tubs and saunas, can be destructive during pregnancy. Limit time in these conditions to forestall overheating.

- Be Wary of Lifting:

Abstain from truly difficult work or demanding exercises that could strain your body. Lift with your legs as opposed to your back to forestall superfluous pressure.

- Try not to skip dinners.Keep up with ordinary feasts to guarantee a reliable admission of supplements. Skipping feasts can prompt low glucose levels, influencing both you and the child.

- Limit Upsetting Circumstances:

Limit openness to upsetting circumstances however much could be expected. Practice unwinding methods, like profound breathing or reflection, to successfully oversee pressure.

Continuously talk with your medical services supplier, assuming that you have concerns or inquiries regarding explicit exercises or propensities during pregnancy. Their direction is fundamental to guaranteeing a protected and solid pregnancy for both you and your child.

Practical tips for a safe and healthy pregnancy

A combination of lifestyle decisions, appropriate medical attention, and self-care routines are necessary to ensure a safe and healthy pregnancy. Here are a number of thorough, useful suggestions to help you have a happy pregnancy experience:

1. Prompt and Consistent Prenatal Care:

   As soon as you find out you are pregnant, make an appointment for your first prenatal visit. Frequent examinations are essential for tracking the baby's growth and resolving any possible problems.

2. Balanced Nutrition: Make sure your diet is well-balanced by consuming a range of

fruits, vegetables, whole grains, dairy products, and lean meats. Make sure you are getting enough of the important nutrients, such as calcium, iron, folic acid, and omega-3 fatty acids.

3. Hydration: Throughout the day, make sure you drink lots of water to stay hydrated. Staying properly hydrated helps to maintain the amniotic fluid, avoid dehydration,and facilitate digestion.

4. Regular Exercise: With the consent of your healthcare provider, take part in moderate, low-impact exercises. Exercises that improve both your physical and mental health include swimming, walking, and prenatal yoga.

5. Adequate Rest: Give adequate rest and restorative sleep top priority. To find the most comfortable sleeping position for you, try a variety of positions and use pillows for support.

6. Control Stress: Engage in stress-relieving activities like yoga for pregnant women, meditation, or deep breathing. Excessive levels of stress can be harmful to the baby and to you.

7. Refrain from Hazardous Substances: Refrain from using tobacco, alcohol, and recreational drugs. Reduce your exposure to environmental risks as much as possible, and discuss any worries you have with your healthcare provider.

8. Educate yourself: Attend prenatal classes to learn about lactation, childbirth, and postpartum medical attention. Possessing knowledge lowers anxiety and gives you the ability to make wise decisions.

9. Weight Management: Try to gain weight in a healthy way while staying within the suggested range. Your pre-pregnancy body mass index (BMI) can be used by your healthcare provider to guide you.

10. Appropriate Posture: Be mindful of your posture, particularly when your body changes. Avoid standing or sitting for extended periods of time, and make use of supportive chairs.

11. Oral Health:Observe proper dental hygiene. Regular dental checkups are

crucial because hormonal changes during pregnancy can raise the risk of gum disease.

12. Monitor blood pressure: Pay attention to your pulse rate. Reporting any significant changes to your healthcare provider is important because high blood pressure can cause complications.

13. Steer Clear of High-Risk Activities: Steer clear of anything that could be dangerous. injuries to the abdomen or falling. For information on particular activities that might be risky during pregnancy, speak with your healthcare provider.

14. Schedule Bathroom Breaks: As your child gets older, you might need to go to the bathroom more frequently. To support

bladder control, schedule bathroom breaks and engage in pelvic floor exercises.

15. Create a support system. Get a network of friends, family, and medical professionals who will be there for you. Express your worries and, if necessary, ask for advice.

Recall that each pregnancy is distinct and that every person's needs may differ. See your doctor on a regular basis to discuss any concerns you may have and to make sure your pregnancy is safe and healthy.

Prenatal Care and Testing:

Nurturing a Healthy Pregnancy

- Go for customary pre-birth check-ups:

Plan and go to all suggested pre-birth check-ups. These arrangements are critical for checking both your wellbeing and the child's turn of events.

- Keep a Reasonable Eating Routine:

Focus on organic products, vegetables, entire grains, lean proteins, and dairy to help the child's development.

- Participate in moderate activity:

Partake in customary, moderate activity with your medical care supplier's endorsement. Exercises like strolling, swimming, and pre-birth yoga can advance general prosperity.

- Get Satisfactory Rest:

Guarantee that you get sufficient rest. Pay attention to your body's signs and enjoy reprieves when expected to oversee weakness and diminish pressure.

- Remain Hydrated:

Drink a lot of water to remain hydrated. Appropriate hydration is fundamental for keeping up with amniotic fluid levels and supporting general wellbeing.

- Teach Yourself:

Find out about the various phases of pregnancy, labor, and postpartum care. Go to pre-birth classes to acquire important information and plan for the impending changes.

- Practise great cleanliness.

Keep up with great individual cleanliness by cleaning up routinely. This lessens the risk of diseases that can affect both you and the child.

- Wear Open to Apparel:

Choose a dress that suits your evolving body. Strong shoes can lighten distress and decrease the burden on your back and feet.

Keep in mind that each pregnancy is extraordinary, so it's vital to tailor these dos to your singular necessities. Standard correspondence with your medical services supplier guarantees customised direction and a smoother pregnancy venture

Chapter4

Guiding Your Health Through Pregnancy:

Monitoring vital signs and addressing concerns

Vital sign monitoring is essential during pregnancy to protect the developing baby's health as well as the mother's. The following are important vital signs to monitor:

Blood Pressure (BP): Check your blood pressure on a regular basis. Systolic <120 mm Hg and diastolic <80 mm Hg define the normal range. High blood pressure can cause problems, like preeclampsia.

Heart Rate (HR): Keep a regular eye on your heart rate. 60 to 100 beats per minute is the normal range. An elevated heart rate could be a sign of stress or other issues. Breaths per minute are used to calculate the respiratory rate (RR). 12 to 20 breaths per minute is the normal range. Investigations into abnormal respiratory rates might be necessary.

Body temperature: it should be taken on a regular basis. The standard range is 36-37.2°C (97-99°F). High temperatures could be a sign of an infection or other problems.

Weight: Track your weight increase in accordance with medical advice. Is it normal to gain weight steadily and gradually during a healthy pregnancy?

Fetal Movement: Observe how the infant moves. Notify your healthcare provider of any notable adjustments or decreases in activity.

Blood Tests: To keep an eye on a number of indicators, do as prescribed by your doctor. Tests for iron, blood sugar, and blood count may be performed.

Urinary Output: Track the amount of urine produced. Sufficient production is necessary; deviations could point to possible problems.

Glycemic Management: If gestational diabetes is detected, control blood sugar levels. Dietary management and routine observation are crucial.

A successful and healthy pregnancy is largely dependent on keeping an eye on these crucial markers and keeping lines of communication open with medical professionals. For tailored care, always heed the advice and suggestions given by your medical team. Attend prenatal checkups on time to consult with a healthcare provider and report any odd

Common pregnancy symptoms and management

A woman's life is transformed during pregnancy, bringing with it a variety of physical and hormonal changes. Comprehending and handling typical symptoms is essential for a safe pregnancy. The following list of common symptoms and helpful management techniques includes:

Morning sickness:

Symptoms include occasional vomiting and nausea, which usually start in the morning but can last all day.

Management: Consume small, frequent meals; drink peppermint or ginger tea to stay hydrated; think about wearing acupressure wristbands; speak with a doctor about safe anti-nausea drugs.

Fatigue:

Symptoms: Feeling overly exhausted and requiring more sleep than normal.

Management: Make sleep a priority; schedule naps; eat a balanced diet high in foods high in iron; exercise lightly and frequently; let your support system know what you need.

Tenderness in the Breasts:

Signs: enhanced susceptibility

as well as breast tenderness.

Management: Use warm compresses for comfort, wear a supportive bra, discuss any concerns with your healthcare provider, and think about applying hypoallergenic creams or ointments.

Frequent urination:

Symptoms: pressure on the bladder and hormonal changes that cause frequent urges to urinate.

Management: Drink plenty of water, go to the bathroom frequently, work on your pelvic floor, cut back on caffeine, and let your doctor know if you experience any pain or discomfort.

Constipation:

Symptoms: Difficulty passing stools, frequently brought on by hormonal fluctuations that impact the digestive tract.

Management: Eat foods high in fibre, drink plenty of water, exercise gently on a regular basis, and talk to your doctor about safe laxative options.

Mood swings:

Symptoms: Hormonal changes causing an emotional swing

Management: Share your emotions with your network of support; think about doing yoga or meditation during pregnancy.

for mental health; if excessive mood swings occur, get expert assistance.

Indigestion and heartburn:

Symptoms: chest burning, frequently after eating.

Management: Sit up straight after eating; avoid acidic and spicy foods; eat smaller, more frequent meals; ask your doctor about safe antacids.

It's important to keep in mind that each pregnancy is different and that people's experiences can differ. Prenatal visits with your doctor on a regular basis guarantee individualized advice and assistance. For a safe and comfortable pregnancy experience, don't be afraid to consult a professional if you have questions or notice severe symptoms.

Kindly seek the advice of a healthcare professional tailored to your individual circumstances

Exercise during pregnancy

Exercise is advantageous during pregnancy, advancing physical and mental prosperity for both the mother and child. Notwithstanding, it's crucial to approach it with alertness and adhere to rules to guarantee wellbeing. Here are some central issues to consider:

Talk with Your Medical Services Supplier:

Prior to beginning or proceeding with a work-out daily practice, counsel your medical services supplier to guarantee it's safe for your singular wellbeing and pregnancy.

Pick safe exercises:

Decide on low-influence activities like strolling, swimming, fixed cycling, or pre-birth yoga. These exercises are delicate on the joints and lessen the risk of injury.

Pay attention to your body.

Focus on how your body works out. Assuming that you feel any inconvenience, tipsiness, or windiness, pause and rest. Adjust or skip practices that don't feel appropriate for you.

Remain Hydrated and Cool:

Drink a lot of water to remain hydrated, and abstain from overheating. Practice in a very well-ventilated space, wear a free, breathable dress, and pick proper times during the day to stay away from outrageous temperatures.

Pelvic Floor Activities:

Incorporate pelvic floor activities to further develop strength and support for the pelvic district. These activities, like Kegels, can be advantageous during pregnancy and postpartum.

Stay away from high-chance exercise.

Avoid exercises with a high risk of falling or sustaining a stomach injury. Physical games and energetic high-influence practices requiring lying level on your back after the primary trimester ought to be avoided.

posture and body mechanics:

Focus on an appropriate stance while working out. Be aware of body mechanics to forestall stress on your back and joints. Connect with your centre muscles to help your spine.

Pre-birth Classes:

Consider joining pre-birth practice classes led by affirmed teachers. These classes are customized to the necessities of pregnant ladies and have a steady climate.

Post-pregnancy contemplations:

Subsequent to conceiving an offspring, bit by bit move once again into exercise with your medical care supplier's endorsement. Centre around remaking centre strength and tending to any post-pregnancy concerns.

Keep in mind that the objective of activity during pregnancy is to keep up with wellness

Chapter 5:

Trimester Insights and Changes:

Understanding the Three Pregnancy Phases

The main trimester is the earliest period of pregnancy. It begins on the main day of your last period—before you're even really pregnant—and goes on for the rest of the thirteenth week. Knowing what's in store will assist you with preparing for the months to come.

First Trimester Changes in Your Body

Pregnancy is different for each woman. A few ladies shine with great wellbeing during those initial 3 months; others feel totally hopeless. Here are a portion of the progressions you could see, what they mean, and which signs warrant a call to your primary care physician.

- **Bleeding**: Around 25% of pregnant ladies have slight bleeding during their first trimester. From the get-go of the pregnancy, light spotting might be an indication that the prepared, undeveloped organism has embedded in your uterus. Be that as it may, on the off chance that you have serious bleeding, squeezing, or sharp pain. in your stomach, call the specialist. These could be indications of an unsuccessful labor or ectopic pregnancy (a pregnancy wherein the incipient organism inserts beyond the uterus).

- **Sore breasts:** Sore breasts are one of the earliest indications of pregnancy. They're set off by hormonal changes, which are preparing your milk channels to take care of your child. Your breasts will presumably be sore all through the primary trimester. Going up a bra size (or more) and wearing a help bra can cause you to feel more great. You most likely won't return to your normal bra size until after your child is done nursing.

- **Constipation**. During pregnancy, elevated degrees of the chemical progesterone delayed the muscle withdrawals that regularly move food through your framework. Add to that the additional iron you're getting from your pre-birth nutrient, and the outcome is awkward stoppage and gas that can keep you feeling swollen all through your pregnancy. Eat more fibre and drink additional liquids to keep things moving all the more easily. Active work can likewise help.

- **Discharge: It is generally** expected to see a dainty, smooth white release (called leukorrhea) in your pregnancy. You can wear an underwear liner on the off chance that it causes you to feel better, but don't use a tampon since it could place microorganisms in your vagina. In the event that the release smells truly horrible, assuming it's green or yellow, or, on the other hand, assuming there's a great deal of clear release, call the specialist.

- **Weakness**: Your body is striving to help a developing child. Lay down for rest or rest when you really want to during the day. Ensure you're getting sufficient iron.

- **Foods have different preferences**. Despite the fact that you may not need a bowl of mint chip frozen yogurt finished off with dill pickles, as the old generalization goes, your preferences can change while you're pregnant. Over 60% of pregnant women have food desires. The greater part have food sources they truly could do without. Surrendering to desires every once in a while is alright; practise good eating habits.

- **Peeing a great deal**: Your child is still little; however, your uterus is developing and it's coming down on your bladder. Accordingly, you might feel like you need to go to the restroom constantly. Try not to quit drinking liquids; your body needs them; however, cut down on caffeine (which invigorates your bladder), particularly before sleep time. At the point when nature calls, respond to it right away. Try not to hold it in.

- **Heartburn**. During pregnancy, your body delivers a greater amount of the chemical progesterone. It loosens up smooth muscles. These muscles ordinarily hold food and acids down in your stomach. At the point when they relax, you can get heartburn, also called acid reflux. To stay away from the burn. Eat a couple of little meals over the course of the day. Try not to reschedule just after you eat. Stay away from oily, fiery, and acidic food varieties (like citrus organic products). and raising your pillow when you rest.

- **Mood swings**: Expanded weakness and changing chemicals can put you on a profound thrill ride that takes you from glad to hopeless or from confident to unnerved in no time flat. It's alright to cry; however, on the off chance that you feel overpowered, attempt to track down a figured-out ear. You can converse with your accomplice, a companion, a relative, or even an expert.

- **Morning sickness:** nausea is one of the most well-known pregnancy side effects. Up to 85% of pregnant women have it. It results from chemical changes in your body, and it can endure through the whole first trimester. For a few pregnant ladies, sickness is gentle. Others can't begin their day without nausea, which is typically more terrible in the first part of the day (subsequently the name "morning sickness"). To quiet your nausea, have a go at eating little, tasteless, or high-protein snacks and clear natural products like juice (a squeezed apple) or soda. You might need to try and do this before you get up. Keep away from any food varieties that make you sick. Nausea itself is nothing to stress over; however, in the event that it's extreme or simply will not disappear, it can influence how much sustenance your child gets. Call your PCP in the event that you can't quit hurling or can't hold down any food.

- **Weight gain**. Pregnancy is one of only a handful of exceptional times in a lady's life when weight gain is viewed as something to be thankful for, yet don't go overboard. During the main trimester, you ought to gain around 3-6 pounds (your primary care physician might propose you change your weight gain up or down in the event that you began your pregnancy underweight or overweight). In spite of the fact that you're conveying an additional individual, you truly aren't eating for two. You just need about 150 extra calories per day during the principal trimester. Get those calories the right way by adding additional foods grown from the ground, such as milk, whole-grain bread, and lean meat, to your eating routine.

The second trimester changes in your body.

During the second trimester of pregnancy, you may go through the following physical changes:

- **expanding breasts and belly**: Your belly grows as your uterus enlarges to accommodate the growing baby. Your breasts will also continue to enlarge over time. Wearing a bra with wide straps is necessary.
- **contractions of Braxton Hicks**: These gentle, erratic contractions may cause a slight constriction in your abdomen. They are more likely to happen in the late

afternoon or early evening, following exercise or sexual activity. If the contractions become regular and stronger over time, get in touch with your doctor. This might indicate premature labor.

- **Dental problems**: Your gums may become more sensitive to brushing and flossing during pregnancy, which could lead to mild bleeding. Irritation can be reduced by using a softer toothbrush and saltwater rinses. Regular visits may also damage your tooth enamel and increase your risk of cavities. Make sure you continue receiving dental care while expecting

- **lightheadedness**: Circulation changes brought on by pregnancy may make you feel lightheaded. Drink lots of water, avoid standing for extended periods of time, and move carefully when standing up or changing positions if you're experiencing dizziness. Lay on your side if you're feeling lightheaded.

- **Skin tones vary.** Pregnancy-related hormonal changes cause your skin's melanin (pigment-bearing cells) to proliferate. Consequently, you may develop melasma, or brown patches, on your face. Additionally, a dark line (the linea nigra) may be visible down your abdomen. These skin alterations are typical and typically go away after delivery. However, exposure to the sun can make the problem worse. Don't forget to wear sunscreen outside. Additionally, you may observe stretch marks—reddish-brown, black, silver, or purple lines—along your thighs, breasts, buttocks, and abdomen. Stretch marks are unavoidable, but most eventually lose their intensity.

- **Nasal problems:** Your body produces more blood and more hormones . This can make your mucous membranes swell and bleed more readily, which can cause stuffiness and nosebleeds . Congestion can be relieved with saline drops or a saline rinse. To help hydrate your skin, use a humidifier, drink lots of water, and apply petroleum jelly to the outside corners of your nose.

- **Leg cramps:** As pregnancy goes on, leg cramps become more frequent and usually happen at night. Stretch your calf muscles before bed, maintain an active lifestyle, and consume lots of water to avoid them. Consider support, comfort, and functionality when selecting shoes. Stretch the affected side's calf muscle if you experience a leg cramp. Ice massages, warm baths, and hot showers could also be beneficial.
- **Vaginal discharge:** A sticky, transparent, or white vaginal discharge may be observed. This is typical. If the discharge starts to smell strongly, changes colour, or is accompanied by pain, soreness, or itching in your vaginal region, get in touch with your healthcare provider. This might point to an infection in the vagina.

- **Infections of the urinary tract:** pregnancy is a common time for these infections. If you have a strong, uncontrollable urge to urinate, sharp pain when you do so, cloudy or strongly scented urine, a fever, or a backache, get in touch with your healthcare provider. Kidney infections can develop from urinary tract infections if they are not treated.

Third trimester changes in your body

Your third trimester experiences will be influenced by your body and hormones.

You might experience your initial pregnancy fatigue again. If you can, try to get a good night's sleep and schedule naps.

Throughout this trimester, especially in the beginning, you will feel your baby move. Additionally, you might feel the baby move down in your abdomen.

This could trigger the "nesting instinct." You might feel compelled to finish preparing things for the baby or clean the house. In order to avoid exhausting yourself, go slowly.

As you get ready for labor, delivery, and parenthood, you might experience increased emotions.

During this trimester, your body might go through certain physical changes.

Puffiness and swelling:

Retention of fluid and The reason for the swelling in your hands, face, ankles, feet, and legs is slowed blood circulation.

Please contact your physician if the swelling in your hands and face gets severe. In addition, if you experience headaches, blurred vision, dizziness, or stomach pain, contact your doctor right away. These could be indicators of preeclampsia, a potentially fatal illness.

Both numbness and tingling:

Your body's swelling may put pressure on nearby nerves, resulting in tingling and numbness. It can occur in your hands, arms, and legs. Your belly's skin may feel so stretched out that it becomes numb.

The most common cause of tingling and numbness in the hands is carpal tunnel syndrome. That is brought on by pressure on a wrist nerve. Maybe you can get rid of these signs by sleeping with wrist splints on. Usually, the issue gets better after pregnancy.

Reflux:

a sour taste in the mouth and throat and a burning sensation in the lower chest.

veins that vary:

These are veins beneath the skin's surface that are blue in colour, swollen, and occasionally painful. They frequently appear on the inside of the legs or the backs of the calves.

The pressure your developing uterus places on the large veins behind it slows blood circulation, which is the cause of varicose veins.

hips, pelvis, and back aches:

It's possible that this began in the second trimester. Your growing belly will put more strain on your back. Pregnancy hormones cause the joints between your pelvic bones to relax, preparing your hips and pelvic area for childbirth. Using a pillow behind your back while you sleep could ease your back pain.

stomach ache:

The tough, rope-like bands of tissue that support the uterus in your belly, called ligaments and muscles, will keep stretching as your baby grows. They might hurt.

Breathing difficulties:

Your lungs' capacity to expand for breathing will decrease as your uterus grows larger.

Increased breast expansion: It's possible that your nipples are tender and secrete colostrum, a yellowish liquid. This liquid will be your baby's first meal if you breastfeed.

Gaining weight:

It is likely that you will gain weight at the start of your third trimester. As delivery draws near, your weight should stabilize.

Discharge from the vagina:

The discharge might go up. Contact your doctor immediately if you notice any blood or if fluid is leaking.

stretches marks:

Your skin will gradually become more stretched as the baby grows. Stretch marks could result from this. These may appear as tiny wrinkles on your skin. They frequently show up on your thighs, breasts, and stomach.

Reduced movement of the fetus:

Your unborn child will eventually outgrow the space in your uterus as they grow larger. You may notice fewer movements during the day as a result. Give your doctor a call if you're worried about your inability to move.

Complications of pregnancy

Pregnancy is a complex physiological interaction, and keeping in mind that numerous pregnancies progress without difficulties, a few ladies might encounter difficulties that require clinical consideration. It's critical to take note that the data given here is certainly not a substitute for proficient clinical guidance. Continuously talk with a medical services supplier for customized direction. Here are a few likely complexities of pregnancy:

**1. Unnatural birth cycle:

Characterized as the departure of a pregnancy before the twentieth week, unsuccessful labors are generally normal and frequently happen because of chromosomal irregularities.

**2. Ectopic Pregnancy:It happens when the prepared egg inserts outside the uterus, as a rule in the fallopian tube. This is a health-related crisis as it can prompt a burst and inside death.

**3. Gestational Diabetes:

A few ladies develop diabetes during pregnancy, which influences glucose levels. Legitimate administration is vital to forestall intricacies for both the mother and child.

**4. Preterm Birth:

It is referred to as a preterm to deliver the child before 37 weeks of growth. The child may experience medical issues as a result of delayed healing following preterm birth.

**5. Toxemia: A potentially problematic ailment characterized by hypertension and organ damage, usually to the kidneys and liver. Usually, it occurs after 20 weeks of pregnancy.

**6. Placenta Previa: This condition can result in draining and may necessitate a caesarean section for delivery because the placenta or completely covers the cervix.

**7. Placental Suddenness: Before delivery, the placenta separates from the uterine wall, which causes death. It is usually a health-related crisis that needs to be briefly mediated.

**8. Intrauterine Growth Restriction (IUGR): If a child isn't developing at a normal pace,there might be a placenta issue or other issues affecting the development of the fetus.

**9. Gestational hypertension: This type of hypertension develops during pregnancy but does not show up in toxemia models. To avoid misunderstandings.

**10. Various Incubation Difficulties: Preterm birth and low birth weight are associated with increased chances of twins, trios, or higher-request products.

**11. Gestational Thyroid Issues: Unbalanced thyroid chemical traits during pregnancy can impact the course of the fetus and may need monitoring and medication.

**12. Rh Contrariness: a condition in which the mother's blood's Rh component conflicts with the child's blood, potentially causing the infant to become homolytically ill.

**13. Hyperemesis Gravidarum: Extreme vomiting and queasiness during pregnancy, which causes dehydration and weight loss.

**14. Profound Vein Apoplexy (DVT): Pregnant women are more likely to develop blood clots, especially in the legs, which can be dangerous if they go to the lungs. This condition requires clinical intervention to monitor side effects.

**15. Weight and Overweight: Being overweight increases the risk of gestational diabetes, hypertension, and caesarean delivery, among other complications.

**16. Contaminations: Both the mother and the unborn child may be at risk from pregnancy-related contaminants such as urinary tract infections or physical contaminants.

Chapter 6

Labor and Delivery:
Final stages of pregnancy

The final phase refers to the early postpartum period and the minutes leading up to the introduction of your child. This is a serious and active stage that involves administering the placenta and actually delivering the child. This guide will help you explore these final stages:

**1. Change and Pushing: Change represents the advancement from the first and second stages of labor and is the point at which the cervix is fully enlarged (10 centimetres).

There may be strong urges to push during this phase. To truly push, pay attention to your body's cues and collaborate with your medical services team.

**2. Pushing Techniques: Follow the advice of your healthcare provider regarding the appropriate time and manner of pushing.

Pushing typically occurs during withdrawals, and you may feel pressure to push through as if you were having a bowel movement.

**3. Solace and Support: Your partner, family, or a doula, along with your introduction to the global support network, can provide local assistance and support during this severe phase.

**4. Episiotomy and Perineal Consideration: In order to assist with conveyance, an episiotomy—a precise cut to lengthen the vaginal opening—may occasionally be carried out. Perineal care is important for promoting recovery following delivery.

**5. Child's Head Arises: The child's head will start to rise as you apply pressure. We call this delegated. Your healthcare provider will advise you on when to push for controlled conveyance and when to take a break.

6. Conveyance of the Child: The child's entire body follows the head in conveying. The person providing your medical care will oversee the movement of your body and shoulders.

**7. Prompt Skin-to-Skin Contact: When circumstances permit, make prompt skin-to-skin contact with the child. This promotes soothing and temperature control for the child.

**8. Postponed Line Bracing: Discuss with your healthcare provider the option of deferred line bracing, which gives the baby more time to receive blood from the placenta.

**9. Placenta Conveyance: The placenta needs to be conveyed after the baby is conceived. Compared to the earlier stages, this one is typically less severe and more constrained.

**10. Uterine back rub: This procedure may be carried out by your medical services provider.

aid in uterine contraction and reduce the likelihood of postpartum discharge.

**11. Postpartum Checks: When the placenta is delivered, your healthcare provider will check it for cuts or rips and make any necessary repairs. Vaginal and perineal examinations are routine.

**12. Initial Child Assessments: The medical services group will oversee the child's initial assessments, which will include estimations, Apgar scores, and overall prosperity.

**13. Breastfeeding Commencement: If you plan to nurse your child, the initial care may begin shortly after delivery. It can be beneficial to receive assistance from healthcare providers or lactation consultants.

**14. Recovery following pregnancy: You will proceed to the post-pregnancy recovery area following the conveyance. This is a time to relax and adhere.

Chapter 7

Postpartum Care:

Strategies for self-care

The physical strain of pregnancy, labor, and delivery is great. Even though it might be easier said than done, getting enough sleep is crucial for promoting your body's ability to heal.

Take a nap yourself, or ask a friend or family member to watch your child while you get some rest.

Take advantage of the time to unwind, even if you don't sleep when your baby naps.

Take your time, even though you might be itching to return to your pre-baby figure.

Steer clear of crash diets, especially if you are nursing and in need of the additional calories and nutrients.

After giving birth, it's crucial to stay active, but before starting any more demanding exercise than walking,

Consult your doctor. Make sure your diet is balanced with plenty of fruits, vegetables, and eggs.

Consult your doctor if you have any dietary restrictions, as they may impact your vitamin content or milk supply, and determine whether you need to take any supplements.

Newborn care basics

Congratulations on the birth of your precious child! Feeling a mixture of excitement and perhaps a hint of anxiety as you embark on this amazing journey of parenthood is normal. The message is intended to guide you through the basic principles of caring for a newborn, providing you with useful information and guidance to ensure a happy and uneventful beginning.

1. Breastfeeding and bottlefeeding

Welcome to the art of nursing. As you and your child together explore this growing experience, make sure the lock is agreeable and have patience. An enjoyable breastfeeding experience can be achieved by creating a daily schedule and recognizing and attending to signs.

Bottle Feeding: If you decide to bottle feed your child, make sure the recipe meets their nutritional needs. Observe appropriate disinfection.

2. Diapering:

Diaper changes will become a continuous part of your daily practice. Keep a load of diapers, wipes, and diaper rash cream convenient. Guarantee that the diaper is cozy yet not excessively close, and clean the diaper region delicately to forestall aggravation.

3. Rest:

Babies rest a great deal; however, their rest is much of the time; in short, they explode. Establish a comfortable rest climate, wrap up your child in the event that they appreciate it, and lay out a sleep time routine to flag when now is the ideal time to rest. Show restraint; examples of rest will develop after some time.

4.Cleaning:

Taking a shower can be an excellent experience. Make use of a mild, fragrance-free child cleanser. When your child is taking a shower, support their head and neck and make sure the water is just warm enough. Make taking a shower enjoyable and relaxing.

5. Clothing:

Dress your infant in delicate, breathable attire. Check for indications of overheating or distress, and remember that infants are more happy with being marginally hotter than adults. Keep caps on in a cooler climate to hold body heat.

6. Holding:

I love the snapshots of you holding your child. Participate in skin-to-skin contact, sing bedtime songs, and converse with your child. These corporations encourage serious areas of strength for an association and add to your child's general prosperity.

7. Paediatrician Visits:

Standard check-ups with your paediatrician are essential. Monitor development achievements, immunizations, and any worries you might have. Make it a point to ask questions—your paediatrician is an important asset for direction.

8. Perceiving Signals:

Figure out how to decipher your child's signals. Whether it's yearning, sluggishness, or distress, understanding your child's signs will assist you with answering instantly to their requirements, reinforcing the parent-kid bond.

9. Show restraint toward yourself:

Nurturing is an excursion into development and variation. Show restraint toward yourself as you explore the difficulties and delights of really focusing on your infant. Pay attention to your gut feelings, and remember that each child is special.

10.Rest on Help:

Encircle yourself with an encouraging group of people. Companions, family, and different guardians can offer guidance, consolation, and a listening ear when required. Life as a parent is a common encounter, and you're in good company on this staggering excursion.

Embrace every second, and relish in the adoration and euphoria that your infant brings into your life. You're leaving on a wonderful experience, and as time passes, you'll observe the surprising development and improvement of your little one.

I wish you perpetual delight, love, and remarkable minutes in this exceptional section of being a parent.

Infant illnesses

Infants can be susceptible to various illnesses. Common ones include:

1. Respiratory Infections: such as the common cold, flu, or bronchiolitis.
2. Gastrointestinal infections include diarrhea and vomiting caused by viruses or bacteria.
3. Ear Infections: Otitis media is a common ailment among infants.
4. Fever is often a sign of an underlying infection.
5. Rashes: conditions like diaper rash, eczema, or viral rashes.
6. Allergies: Certain foods or environmental elements may cause allergies in some infants.
7. Jaundice: yellowing of the skin or eyes due to elevated bilirubin levels.
8. Urinary Tract Infections (UTIs): Less common but can occur.

It's crucial to consult a healthcare professional if you notice any concerning symptoms in your infant, as their immune systems are still developing. Regular check-ups and vaccinations also play a vital role in preventing certain illnesses.

Chapter 8

Emotional adjustment:

Recognizing postpartum depression and seeking support

A new baby's birth can cause a wide range of emotional changes. A lot of women experience a brief period of mild depression after giving birth. It's important to distinguish between postnatal depression, which is far more severe and typically lasts for a longer period of time, and postnatal "blues," or feeling down. You might have a term for the "blues" or mild depression that women go through after giving birth. When talking about this subject with women and their families, use this term to set it apart from postpartum depression, which is something entirely different.

The mother may have postnatal depression if she feels lethargic, has trouble sleeping or eating, or has low energy. blues. When a woman experiences significant depression that lasts longer than two weeks and interferes with her daily activities, it is considered true postnatal depression. She might additionally encounter any of the following:

- persistent melancholy, anxiety, or agitation
- low enjoyment of or interest in once-enjoyable activities
- challenges of completing daily tasks at work, school, home, or in social situations
- Feelings of hopelessness or negativity toward herself or her baby
- multiple symptoms (aches, pains, palpitations, and numbness) with no apparent physical cause, as well as depressing or hopeless feelings about herself or her newborn.

She might also be experiencing guilt or harbouring unfavourable thoughts about her newborn or herself. A woman may occasionally experience such severe depression that she considers suicide. If a newlywed mother exhibits signs of depression, you should refer her as quickly as possible to the closest medical establishment. Support networks can be beneficial as well. Should that prove unfeasible, you might have to provide for her during this time. Meet with her frequently, if at all possible, and make use of your abilities to empathize with her, listen to her, and offer support. Get her permission to talk to a friend or family member who she believes could also be able to help her. Get her involved in social events and past pursuits that brought her joy. Exercise on a regular basis can be very beneficial for mild depression.

Role of dad's in postpartum

In the post pregnancy period, fathers assume complex parts:

Basic Encouragement: Giving consolation, understanding, and sympathy to the mother as she explores the physical and inner difficulties of post pregnancy recuperation.

Viable Help: Adding to family errands, including cooking, cleaning, and overseeing day to day liabilities, to ease the new mother's responsibility and advance a steady climate.

Childcare Obligations: Effectively taking part in focusing on the infant, for example, diaper changes, taking care of, and mitigating, encouraging a common obligation in nurturing.

Correspondence: Taking part in transparent correspondence to address concerns, share sentiments, and keep serious areas of strength for an association during this groundbreaking period.

Backing: Pushing for the mother's prosperity, guaranteeing she gets the fundamental help, rest, and taking care of oneself to support her recuperation and change in accordance with parenthood.

Holding with the Child: Effectively taking part in holding exercises with the infant, like snuggling, perusing, or playing, to fortify the dad kid relationship.

Consolation: Offering inspirational statements and celebrating little triumphs, recognizing the difficulties and wins of life as a parent

Chapter 9

Parenting:

Parenting Tips and Advice:

Being a parent will challenge all of your limits. These parenting pointers and recommendations might assist you in maintaining an optimistic outlook and approaching particular circumstances with a can-do attitude. Not just your child but also others will grow.

Prepare yourself for the journey:

It's not uncommon for seasoned parents to recall their first year of parenthood as being like riding a rollercoaster. That analogy is very true, as the experience will be exhilarating in every way. It's possible for you to laugh one moment and cry the next. After completing a task, you might feel like a super parent one minute, and the next, you might find yourself searching the internet. You might even be lamenting your former nonparent identity during this whole time. At first, all the changes may seem overwhelming, but you'll quickly get used to it!

Believe in Your Feelings: This proverb, or innumerable variants thereof, has been repeated numerous times before. The manual for raising a child does not exist. Naturally, you could begin reading every book on "good parenting skills" in the hopes of learning some valuable lessons. However, don't assume that you'll enter parenthood unprepared without doing a thorough amount of research. Your natural parenting instincts will take over as soon as you hold your baby, even though you may not be aware of them yet. If, at first, you feel as though you know nothing, don't worry. It's alright to feel that way, but your confidence and parenting abilities will improve with time.

Be patient: Your life will initially seem to revolve around feeding, changing diapers, giving your baby a bath, and comforting them. Be prepared to accomplish all of this with very little sleep! Though it might seem endless, have patience—this state of affairs won't last forever. Even in a few months, as your baby grows, things will change, your routines will change, and your life will look different. Your infant will be a toddler before you know it, and you'll be chasing them all over the house. Additionally, everything will seem to you and them alike like a brand-new adventure. You might feel that way, but your confidence and parenting abilities will improve with time.

Have an open mind: It's not necessary to set yourself up for failure when it comes to becoming or being a parent. No parent is flawless. You are, after all, a human. It's advisable to enter parenthood without preconceived ideas about what or how you should be raising your children. It's risky to step into the chasm between expectation and reality, which can lead to a great deal of worry and anxiety. The secrets to success are to learn to adapt and to keep an open mind! It's not necessary to have solutions for everything, and managing everything at once is not possible. Proceed step-by-step.

Recognize when to Ask for Help: You're not by yourself. You should never be reluctant to ask your friends and family for assistance if you need it. When assistance is needed, your own parents will probably provide it gladly because it will allow them to spend time with their grandchildren. The best part is that, most of the time, best friends, aunts, uncles, and grandparents are more affordable than babysitters! All kidding aside, though, your child will greatly benefit from this bonding experience, as you will be introducing them to people they will eventually grow up with. Asking a friend to pick up some groceries is a simple way to ask for assistance. or give your child to their grandparents, run an errand, or do anything else to give yourself a few hours of much-needed alone time.

Remind yourself that phases will pass as well: A child's life is filled with behavioural phases and stages. Remind yourself that these stages are normal and part of your child's growth. Children start learning and honing their communication skills at this age. Toddlers frequently have tantrums and outbursts because they find it so difficult to express their emotions. Assist your child in verbally expressing their emotions—a skill that requires practice—and establish some fair guidelines and boundaries, upholding them consistently while consistently rewarding good

Communicate: When you are free to spend time with your child, a good book and some coffee or tea go straight out the window. But it's important to reserve a portion of your particularly cherished plans for your own growth. For instance, have a friend, relative, or helper watch the child while you practise yoga for 20 minutes. Once more, if you wait a long time and your child creates, you'll lose more opportunities to present your most trustworthy schedules, and your wrinkles will reappear!

Don't compare: Every child is unique and different from the next. You'll see this in your own children as well as when you become a parent to more kids. Every child is unique in their temperament; some are gregarious, while others are reticent. You might be dealing with a laid-back or boisterous infant. Every child will have a different activity level and manner of adjusting to circumstances. Therefore, it isn't about having a "good" or "bad" child. Accept your child for who they are and learn to work with their temperament (and developmental pace) rather than against it, instead of comparing them to other people's kids!

Lead by example: Consider the exemplary people in your past: Who did they represent? Perhaps they were your parents. Use this chance to set an example for your child. Younger kids imitate everything because they are impressionable. Set an example of selflessness, kindness, tolerance, honesty, and respect. In this case, the adage "treat others the way you want to be treated" is extremely applicable.

Engage in cooperative play: Playing with your child not only helps them learn many different skills but also demonstrates your love for them.

For infants and early children, play is essential for learning and brain development, as well as for fostering strong interpersonal bonds. Playing with you can help your child develop social-emotional skills that will boost their confidence and sense of self-worth.

Examine in accordance with: It's not necessary to have grown up with Examining Rainbow to understand the importance of examining children. It's never too early to begin closely reading books with your child, even if you start early. Examining your child regularly fosters their language and motor skills. Examining them and having consistent conversations with them can have a significant impact on their growth. Furthermore, it will only benefit them in the long run.

Remember Your Own Childhood Years: When you become a parent, a lot of memories from your own upbringing may resurface, including some awful ones you may not have thought about in a while. This is a fantastic opportunity to reflect on them. Think about your upbringing with your people. Perhaps there are a few (or a ton) of things you would do differently with your own child. However, now that you're a parent, there might be some notable customs or practices that you should continue to be aware of.

Value Your Connection: Really focusing on a child can have a negative effect on your assistant-assistant dynamic. It's not unusual for inexperienced parents to miss your life together before having kids. Additionally, you might begin to notice that you and your partner have differing opinions about sustaining, and that's okay. Keep the lines of communication open and collaborate to determine the best course of action and the supporting strategies or techniques that you both find most appealing. Be gentle with one another and set aside a short while for a night on the town. Ask a friend, relative, or babysitter to watch your child if you are unable to do so so that you and your helper can spend quality time together.

Take Care of Yourself: You might discover that taking care of yourself is part of being a second parent. Regularly taking care of oneself by scheduling activities such as yoga. When you are free to spend time with your child, a good book and some coffee or tea go straight out the window. But it's important to reserve a portion of your particularly cherished plans for your own growth. For instance, have a friend, relative, or helper watch the child while you practise yoga for 20 minutes. Once more, if you wait a long time and your child creates, you'll lose more opportunities to present your most trustworthy schedules, and your wrinkles will reappear!

Bonus.

Knowing the warning signs and symptoms of issues that arise after delivery

- Heavy bleeding

- Infection

- High blood pressure

- Heart failure

- Blood clots

- Depression

1.Heavy bleeding

After giving birth, most women experience some vaginal bleeding for two to six weeks. Even after having a caesarean section (C-section), this is still possible. At first, the bleeding may be slightly more intense than a menstrual flow and may include tiny clumps (clots). Every day, normal bleeding should gradually decrease.

It's normal to experience more cramps and possibly more bleeding when breastfeeding, though. Breastfeeding stimulates your body to release certain hormones that help your uterus contract and shrink. Eventually, your menstrual cycle will also resume. If your bleeding completely stops and then resumes. It could be your first period around or after six weeks after giving birth.

Postpartum haemorrhage is the term for excessive bleeding (PPH). Infections, poorly contracted uterus postpartum, and placenta fragments that were not delivered can all result in heavy bleeding. Without emergency care, PPH is a medical emergency that can result in serious illness or even death.

If you experience bleeding that way, get emergency care if bleeding:

- fills a pad and then some every hour.
- continues for three or four days without slowing down.

- soon after delivery, slows down, then becomes heavier or bright red.

- is coupled with excruciating pain or cramps

2. Infection

Skin rips or stitches may be required for C-section incisions after giving birth. Care instructions from your physician for these injuries will be given. However, despite your best efforts, a wound can still get infected.

Antibiotics can treat infections if they are discovered early. Infections have a quick worsening and can even become fatal if left untreated.

Get help right away if you have:

- Clammy or sweaty skin chills
- discharge from the area of the wound.
- severe or worsening discomfort.
- rapid heartbeat or breathing
- fever of at least 100.4 degrees
- Redness around the area of the wound
- Warmth radiates from the wound site.

3. High blood pressure

After giving birth, high blood pressure is referred to as postpartum preeclampsia. The majority of cases happen 48 hours after delivery. However, hypertension can appear up to six weeks following childbirth.

Preeclampsia following childbirth is a medical emergency. If untreated, it may result in seizures, harm to the liver and kidneys, and even death.

Get help right away if you have:

- Reduced need to urinate
- High blood pressure, measured at 140/90 mm Hg or above
- discomfort in the shoulder or upper right abdomen
- severe headaches
- Unexpected weight increase
- Legs, hands, or face swelling
- Breathing difficulties
- Variations in vision, such as bright spots or long-lasting shadows

4. Heart Failure

The heart may become weaker during or soon after pregnancy due to a rare form of heart failure. It is difficult for the body to pump blood when it has peripartum cardiomyopathy.

The heart pumps up to 50% more blood during a healthy pregnancy to support the developing fetus. It is unknown what specifically causes peripartum cardiomyopathy. However, the additional cardiac strain in pregnancy could be a factor. High blood pressure, obesity, diabetes, smoking, being older than 30, and having twins or more are known risk factors for peripartum cardiomyopathy.

Get help right away if you have:

- chest ache
- Overwhelming exhaustion
- accelerated heart rate
- Breathing difficulties
- swelling around the ankles or feet

5. Blood Clots

When a blood clot obstructs a lung artery, it can cause a pulmonary embolism. Clots are one of the most common causes of maternal death, despite their rarity. Blood clots frequently move from the legs to the lungs. Therefore, it's critical to identify the symptoms of leg blood clots.

Following childbirth, some women are more susceptible to blood clots, including those who possess high blood pressure, have undergone a C-section, are obese, or are older than 35. You might be advised by your physician to put on compression stockings as soon as you give birth. After delivery, you might also need to wear them for a few weeks or months.

Get help right away if you have:

- a painfully swollen, red leg that feels warm to the touch.
- chest ache
- breathing heavily or coughing
- Breathing difficulties

6. Severe depression

It's common to experience short-term postpartum depression or tears for a few weeks. However, postpartum depression, a severe form of depression that can last for a long time, affects 10% to 20% of women. Taking care of yourself and your child may be difficult due to the symptoms. These strong emotions are not your fault; assistance is on hand. You will start to feel more like yourself with medicine and counselling.

Get help right away if you have:

- Extreme anger or irritability
- excessive drowsiness or insomnia.
- Lack of enthusiasm for activities you once enjoyed
- Sadness and the desire to cry a lot
- Feeling of helplessness or terror
- extreme fluctuations in mood
- difficulty concentrating or recalling detail

Conclusion

As we close the parts of **"Things to consider while expecting"**.I expand my ardent congrats on arriving at this vital guide in your excursion toward parenthood. Darla B. Humphrey made this aid with a mix of skill and compassion, intending to be a relentless friend as you explore the complexities of pregnancy.

As you ponder the bits of knowledge shared inside these pages, recall that each word is a demonstration of the strength and flexibility inside you. The difficulties and delights of anticipating labor are essentially as exceptional as your singular experience. Embrace the information acquired, love the snapshots of expectation, and have confidence in your capacity to beat difficulties with beauty.

As your process unfolds, may this guide keep on filling in as a wellspring of solace, direction, and motivation. May you track down comfort in the common stories, strengthening in the functional tips, and a feeling of local area, realising that others have strolled in a comparative way.

I wish you a solid and blissful pregnancy, smoothers labor insight, and the boundless joy that accompanies inviting your little one into the world. May the illustrations advanced inside these pages go with you into the experience of being a parent.

With warm respects,

Darla B. Humphrey

www.ingramcontent.com/pod-product-compliance
Lightning Source LLC
Chambersburg PA
CBHW051308250726

48656CB00004B/1543